WAISTLESS

How to Transform Your Waist in 30 Days!

30 Day Meal and Exercise Plan

Abby Ayoola

Published by Abby Ayoola

Disclaimer: The author and publisher shall have no liability or responsibility to any person or entity regarding any loss or damage incurred, or alleged to have incurred, directly or indirectly, by the information contained in this book. This book has been written for information and inspiration only and does not contain all information on the subject of weight-loss, health and fitness.

Always consult your physician before beginning this, or any exercise program. This general information is not intended to diagnose any medical condition or to replace your healthcare professional. Consult with your healthcare professional to design an appropriate exercise prescription. If you experience any pain or difficulty with these exercises, stop and consult your healthcare provider.

ISBN: 978-0-9959104-0-9

DEDICATION

I dedicate this book to all the women out there who are trying to be a better version of themselves. An extra special thanks to my kids, my fiancé, and my family.

I would also like to thank my former bosses that had fired me. If I didn't get fired, I would have remained in a cycle of looking for employment, and would have never started my own business.

I grew up thinking I needed to be in the workforce to make it in life, but with each passing day, I realize that chasing one's dream is the only way to go.

The two most powerful warriors are patience and time.

Leo Tolstoy

'*I Am Ready*' is a poem that I recite to myself every morning for affirmations. I look at my self in the mirror and recite the poem. it gives me clarification, motivation and elevates my mood. I hope it will do the same for you.

I am Ready

I am ready to be a success.
I am ready to fulfil my destiny.
I am ready to become wealthy.
I am no longer scared of the attention that I get.
I am no longer scared of been successful.
I have been through thick and thin and I deserve to be successful.
I deserve to live the life that I want.

ABBY AYOOLA

CONTENTS

Education is the most powerful weapon which you can use to change the world.

NELSON MANDELA

CHAPTER 1
Humble Beginnings

I was born in Nigeria in the mid-80s to a hotel manager and a university student. I grew up in Sagamu, Ogun State, and I remember visiting my dad at the hotel where he managed, which is located in Sagamu. His wife and kids lived in Lagos. Whenever my brother, sisters, and stepmom came to town, my mom would take me to spend some time with them. I remember always going up and down the stairs to deliver fried plantains and eggs to my dad in his office. My dad's office was located on the main floor of the hotel, and we usually stayed on the second floor. We would spend the day together, and when my brother, sisters, and stepmom left for Lagos, my mom would come for me and take me home.

All this went on until the age of eight, at which time I visited my dad in Lagos and enjoyed my time there so much that I asked if I could live there with him and my siblings. They agreed, and I started living with my dad at the age of nine. I remember celebrating my tenth birthday with my classmates in school. Back then, they used to sing for you, let you cut the cake in the classroom and celebrate. After that year, I went to a boarding school called Mayflower in Sagamu with my brother and one of my sisters. I am not even sure if the school still exists. The educational system in Nigeria is faster than the one in North America, so by the age of eleven, I was already in JS1, which is equivalent to grade eight in Canada.

Boarding school was tough, but it taught me how to be disciplined and the importance of exercise and fitness at a young age. They woke us up at 6:00 a.m. to go for a jog for forty-five minutes, then we got about fifteen minutes to shower and get dressed for school. I remember the water being so cold that I had to kneel down to shower so I could tolerate the coldness of the water. We all showered in an open field, so there was no such thing as privacy. We had a girls' hostel and a boys' hostel, so the girls were separated from the boys when it came to showering and getting dressed. After we were dressed, our next step was to go to the cafeteria to eat our breakfast. After breakfast, we had to walk to school for another thirty minutes. So in the morning alone we exercised for over an hour. This was our routine every weekday. On weekends, it was more relaxed. We were allowed visitors, so my mom and stepmom came to visit whenever it was visitation time. In the night time, all the students gathered outside around the stage. We called it social night, as people would perform on stage, dancing, acting out a play, singing, and so on. I enjoyed social night very much. That was usually the highlight of my week.

One day during visitation day, when I was in JS2 almost in JS3, I was told that we would be travelling to Canada that week and should tell no one, so the school administration wouldn't stop us from going. Like 'play-play', we left the hostel, taking only some clothes with us and left everything else. I travelled with my stepmom's brother, his son, my two sisters, and my brother.

When we got to Canada, I had to start from grade seven, because they went by age and not by your academic level. So I did grade seven and grade eight again, even though I had already completed them in Nigeria. Middle school in Canada was a culture shock for me. I was introduced to so many cultures, like Jamaican, Spanish, Ghanaian, Canadian, Vietnamese, and many more. I was bullied by one boy because he claimed I was ugly and had big lips. I never let his words get to me, because he himself wasn't good looking. Then I got into a fight with another boy, but none of those incidents scared me. They were just growing pains and incidents that I learned from.

Any time women come together with a collective intention, it's a powerful thing. Whether it's sitting down making a quilt, in a kitchen preparing a meal, in a club reading the same book, or around the table playing cards, or planning a birthday party, when women come together with a collective intention, magic happens.

PHYLICIA RASHAD

CHAPTER 2
Growing Pains

Growing up, I was always taught that going to university, getting good grades, and choosing a career that will allow you to make lots of money is the ideal way to live. In a Nigerian household, if you are not studying to be a doctor, lawyer, or an engineer, you are a failure. However, I was not interested in any of those career choices. After all, I am a social introvert, if that makes sense. I was more interested in being a model. I liked the camera, and I didn't see myself doing those other jobs for the rest of my life. High school was fun. I went to West Humber Collegiate Institute for grades nine and ten, then we moved to Brampton, and I went to Turner Fenton Secondary School for grades eleven and twelve. Most of my friends went to a local Catholic school.

I didn't start going to nightclubs until grade eleven, but for Nigerian parents that wasn't allowed, so I found creative ways to sneak out or just tell them I was going to work. I got in trouble with my parents growing up, because I always wanted to do things my way and have some fun. I was pretty much labelled the black sheep of the family. I was never a heavy drinker, because I didn't like the taste of alcohol. So in those days, if I had to drink anything, I usually went for Smirnoff Ice. I enjoyed going to all-age jams, tried getting into nineteen-and-over clubs with my fake I.D., and sometimes it worked, sometimes it didn't. I must say for the amount of partying that I did, I never overdid the drinking. I didn't do drugs, and I wasn't reckless either. I valued myself, and I knew that I wanted more from life, but just didn't know how to go about it. I started modelling here and there, did a couple of videos for local artists, an album cover, and some prints.

I was working two jobs and going to high school. I worked at Siblings, which is a clothing retail store for kids, and Cineplex Odeon, a movie theatre. On weekends, I usually had to work both jobs and still find a way to do my homework and assignments. I wasn't an A student or anything, I was more like a B or C student. The only things I got an A in always had to do with food, whether it was a baking class or food and nutrition class. I actually wanted to be a chef right after high school, because I wanted to get paid to travel and eat. I went on a field trip to George Brown College with my classmates to check out the culinary program that they have. However, I left the field trip thinking to myself that I did not want to be wearing a white chef uniform for the rest of my life and be cooped up in a kitchen for long hours, so I scrapped the chef idea.

Then I thought to myself, "I like to be in front of the camera, so why not choose a career that will allow me to be on TV?" So I chose to study 'Journalism: Print and Broadcast' at Canadore College in North Bay. The program wasn't what I expected, because I thought we would be covering events around North Bay, but that wasn't the case. We were sitting in classrooms learning things that had nothing to do with journalism, so I stopped trying and eventually failed my second year of college and dropped out. The ironic part is that I now have my own blog and a cooking show on YouTube. So the two careers that I first chose to study after high school are what I eventually started doing. After dropping out of Canadore College, I went to George Brown to study Human Resources Management, because I was trying to get my CHRP before they changed the rules of becoming one. Then I took online courses to become a nutritionist. I noticed that I always came back to nutrition, so I decided to work in that field, but there aren't many jobs for people like me. The only available options were to become a dietitian aide or work at a restaurant, and I wasn't interested in either of those career choices.

Never give up on what you really want to do. The person with big dreams is more powerful than the one with all the facts.

H JACKSON BROWN, JR.

CHAPTER 3
Getting to Know Myself

While I was at Canadore College studying 'Journalism: Print and Broadcast,' I had lots of fun meeting new people and making decisions on my own with no curfew and no parents breathing down my neck or telling me what to do. I recommend that young people go away for college, because the experience gained from doing so is priceless. I partied almost every night and still made it to my classes in the morning. I remember having snow fights with my roommates and water fights in the house residence. It was truly a memorable and fun time for me. Occasionally, I would get rides from North Bay to Toronto if I had a modelling job to do, or if there was an event that I didn't want to miss.

Growing up, I never had to worry about my weight. I remember one time I was lying down and I felt some fat in my back, let's just say that prompted me to go on my first diet. The cycle started; if I felt like I was getting over my weight range of 135lbs-145lbs, I would go on a diet to bring me back within my range by starving myself. Then when I started eating normally again, I would gain all the weight back, plus more. What I was doing back then was engaging in a vicious cycle of gaining and losing weight. I wasn't educated enough on food and nutrition.

It's about changing your lifestyle to include healthy habits, and not just going on diets. I started learning about healthy foods and implementing them into my diet at the age of twenty-five, which was after college. The only time that I took a course in food and nutrition was in grade ten, three times a week. As a college student, I ate out almost every day, which in turn meant I was consuming lots of sodium and fat, which led to yoyo dieting on my part.

After I had my third baby in 2012, I took an online diploma course in nutrition. I read books, blogs, watched videos, and took on-line courses, all in the name of nutrition. I became a vegan for a whole six months. I gave up chicken, eggs, fish, shrimp, and all other meats. My weight dropped down to 127lbs, which was the lowest I had ever been in my adult life. I loved the way it made me feel—I had energy, and my skin was glowing. But my family and friends told me that I looked like I was suffering, because I was too skinny. I got bored of the vegan lifestyle and started eating meat, again. Within a year, I went from 127lbs to 142lbs. During all my pregnancies, I had always managed to gain 32-40lbs maximum, except for my last pregnancy in 2016 when I only gained 10lbs. I was already 156lbs at the beginning of my 2016 pregnancy, so luckily for me I didn't gain the normal 32-40lbs. The key to staying in shape during pregnancy is to eat the normal portions that you would eat when not pregnant. Don't say, "I am eating for two," because you are not. The nutrients your baby needs get transferred through the umbilical cord, so you do not need to eat extra portions. Go for long walks, and enjoy your pregnancy. Look at it this way, it's only for a short period of time, so enjoy your baby growing inside of you.

In December 2014, I weighed myself and I was 155lbs. I panicked because I had never weighed that much, unless I was pregnant, which I wasn't at the time. That was the moment I chose to take my health into my own hands, yet again, and start working out. The small changes you make today will make a big difference tomorrow.

I played soccer in high school, and that was it. I had worked out maybe ten times in my whole adult life, and over the years the weight crept up on me. So I decided to contact a personal trainer, because I knew if I decided to work out on my own, I wouldn't be consistent enough to make a difference in my health, and wouldn't lose the weight permanently. I started working out with my personal trainer in January 2015, three days per week for a good six months. Then I had to take a break, because something horrible happened in my life in August 2015, and I had to go to court for assault. That was a trying time in my life. I had to move back home with my parents for two months with my three kids at the time. I was checking out properties to rent almost every day, but something always went wrong. They always said, "Why are you looking to move in so fast?" And they wouldn't give the apartment to me. But I thank God that a house became available, and I couldn't have asked for a better house. If it weren't for God and the help of my fiancé and family members, I don't know how I would have survived. My mental health would waver from time to time, and I broke down a couple of times, especially when I was looking for a place to live and all I kept hearing was "No." On top of that, I was in court almost every month, because I had a criminal case, a family court case, and two traffic ticket cases. One thing that was constant in my life at that time was God and the strength He gave me to push through all the hurdles that came my way. I am closer to God now than I have ever been in my life. I try to read the Bible every morning, go to church on Sundays, and just be grateful for the things He has done in my life and the things He is about to do.

This brings me to 2016, when I had my fourth child. So now I have four children to care for and raise, and I take this job very seriously. I strive to be healthy every day so I can be around for my kids, their kids, and so on. After I had my fourth child, within a week I got my pre-pregnancy body back. Everywhere that I went, I was being called the "B-" word, because females couldn't believe that I had just had a baby and already had my flat stomach back. This got me thinking that if I shared the habits that I have accumulated over the years with people, hopefully it would help mothers everywhere and give women hope, whether they are trying to feel sexy, get their pre-pregnancy body back, or trying to lose weight and gain more energy. Let's face it, being pregnant is not the most comfortable thing in the world. Some women get sick, some gain lots of weight, some lose their self-esteem, and some get stretch marks in places they didn't think were possible. I am here to let you know that it is very possible and never too late to gain your confidence, body, health, and your whole purpose in life back. Remember, it is never too late. Change the way you eat, drink, and think about food, and you will not regret it. In the next chapter, I will share with you some tips, tricks, and recipes that I follow in my daily life that have allowed me to gain my body back.

It is never too late to change your life.

ABBY AYOOLA

CHAPTER 4

Tips and Tricks for Weight Loss, Glowing Skin, and Renewed Energy

D rum roll, please. The secret to glowing skin, weight loss, renewed energy, and happiness is food-combining. You may be asking, "What in the hell is food combining?" Food-combining is when you eat certain foods together in a meal to maximize the function of your digestive system. Food-combining is about improving your digestion. It's not about what you eat, it's about what you digest and the nutrients you assimilate into your body. The digestive system's job is to do four things: digest, absorb, assimilate, and eliminate. When we food-combine, we free up more energy to rid our body of free radicals and environmental pollutants, and allow our body to derive the proper nutrients from the food we eat.

Listed below are the rules of food-combining that must be followed:

- Never eat starchy foods with acidic foods in the same meal. Bread, potatoes, pasta, beans, and other carbohydrates should not be eaten together with lemons, oranges, grapefruits, limes, cranberries, or other acid fruits.

- Never eat concentrated proteins and concentrated carbohydrates in the same meal, which means don't mix nuts, meat, eggs, cheese, and other proteins with bread, cereals, pastries, and other carbohydrate foods in one meal.

- Never eat two different concentrated proteins in the same meal. Two proteins of different composition require different concentrations of digestive juices. These juices are not secreted in the stomach at the same time. That is why you should observe the rule of eating only one kind of protein in each meal.

- Don't eat fats with proteins. Cream, butter, sour cream, vegetable oil should not be mixed with meat, eggs, cheese, nuts, or other proteins. Fat suppresses the gastric glands and inhibit the secretion of digestive juices while eating meat, eggs, and nuts.

- Don't eat acidic fruits with proteins. Oranges, lemons, tomatoes, pineapples, cherries, acidic plums, and apples should not be eaten together with meat, nuts, or eggs. The less complicated our food combinations are and the simpler our foods are, the more effective our digestion.

- Don't eat starch with sugar at the same meal. Jellies, jams, fruit butter, sugar molasses, syrups, or bread eaten in one meal with potatoes, sugar, or cereals cause fermentation and poisoning of the body. Usually, feasts with cakes, sweets, pastries lead to vomiting and illness, especially in children and elderly people.

- Eat only one concentrated starch per meal. If two kinds of starch—for example, potatoes and cereal with bread— are eaten in the same meal, one of them will be digested, while the other will lay heavily and untouched in the stomach, it won't pass the intestines and will inhibit other foods from digesting, causing fermentation, increased gastric acidity, belching, and other side effects.

- Don't eat melons with any other foods. Watermelons,

honey melons, cantaloupes, and other kinds of melons should be eaten alone, because melons digest very quickly.

In case you didn't get all of that, I will explain in simpler terms. I have attached a chart to make it easier. Although I have known about food-combining since 2012, I didn't start applying the rules until recently.

The digestive system is a group of organs working together to break down food into energy and nutrients for the entire body. As you can see, the digestive system plays a major role in our health. The digestive system helps us to benefit from the nutrients in our food. If the body doesn't get the proper nutrients, it will start to break down. The burden we give our digestive system is even greater when we consider the modern diet. That's why sometimes after we have eaten a certain type of food, our body shuts down due to all the blood going to the digestive system. We know that raw foods are naturally high in enzymes; for example, fruits and vegetables contain their own plant enzymes that help to aid in digestion. But for the most part, the critical enzymes in modern foods have been destroyed through processing, pasteurization, preserving, and packaging. This means that no matter how healthy and fresh you eat, you may not be digesting

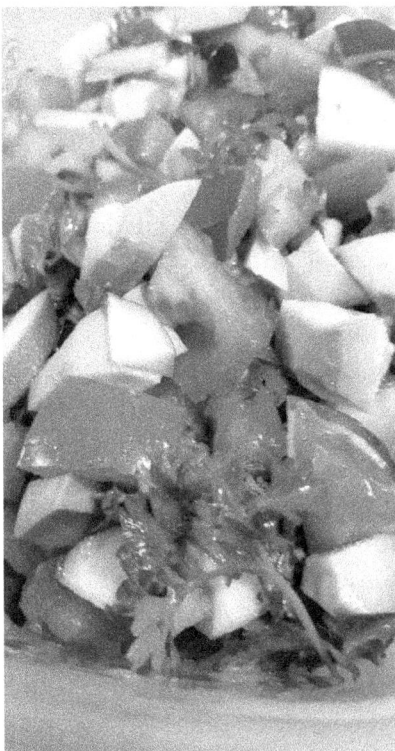

Tomato–Avocado Salad (recipe pg. 43)

and absorbing all the nutrients your body needs without the help of food-combining. You can help your digestion along by eating fermented foods like kimchi and sauerkraut. However, the only thing more important than what we eat is how well we digest it.

It doesn't make sense to eat if your body can't derive any nutrients from it. Proper food-combining is essential to healthy digestion, and the violation of this principle has contributed to the weak digestion, weight gain, imbalanced hormones, and overall ill health we see today. A balanced digestive system has plenty of friendly microflora (good bacteria) and enzymes to help us digest the foods we eat and keep us healthy and strong. The introduction of processed and pasteurized foods, certain drugs, and environmental toxins into our systems has destroyed the natural balance we were created to have. Our modern lifestyle has made conscientious planning and effort a requirement if we want to take care of our digestive system and stay healthy. Learning and practicing the secrets of food-combining is crucial for efficient digestion and better nutrient absorption, which leads to a leaner body, glowing skin, stronger immunity, and increased energy.

WHY FOOD COMBINING WORKS

Different food groups prompt different enzymes to be secreted into the stomach, and each enzyme needs either an acidic or an alkaline environment in which to break down your food. Chemistry tells us that when an acid and an alkali come into contact, they neutralize each other. So, what happens when you eat a food that requires an acidic environment to be broken down and absorbed, together with a food that requires an alkaline environment? Your stomach essentially becomes a neutral zone, neither acidic nor alkaline. This stalls the important work of the enzymes, which inhibits the whole digestive process. When this happens, your food sits in your stomach for too long and begins to ferment and putrefy and form sludge.

The more enzymes you save from digesting food, the more your body is able to ward off sickness, your weight becomes stable, and your skin starts to look better. It also helps to remember that there's a distinct difference between food that ferments in the body and the fermented foods we recommend eating at each meal. Fermented foods, like kimchi, contain beneficial bacteria needed by the gut to support and improve health. Rotting food that ferments in the stomach can become toxic as it moves through the digestive tract.

Fermentation of food promotes alcohol and sugars to be produced. The yeast in your inner digestive system happily feeds off these sugars, multiplying and crowding out the beneficial microflora in your gut, which wreaks havoc on your health. If you already have a weak digestive system or a Candida imbalance, eating improperly combined meals will further weaken your digestive tract, until it slowly begins to break down.

By following the principles of proper food-combining, you will begin to heal your digestive system and allow it to function as it was meant to. You will also experience the following benefits: you will be less bloated after meals, experience no heartburns, and also notice that gas and stomach gurgling are no longer a concern. You may know people with good digestion who can handle meals that are not food-combined properly, but they will often pay the price of digestive discomfort later.

I have provided a system to guide your choice of foods, which makes it easier to decide what to eat. You can use the handy food-combining chart below to make your daily meal decisions both healthy and easy. You will no longer worry about your weight. If you are overweight, you will probably lose weight, because properly combined food is well-assimilated and allows your body to metabolize food better, and more efficient digestion means your body will have more energy left over to work on your hair, skin, and health. I consider food-combining to be another secret to prevent us from aging so quickly. By using food-combining to improve your body's digestion and absorption of nutrients, you will look and feel different. When we follow food-combining, we grow healthier and longer.

That said, it is important for you to understand one overarching concept as we begin. It is a major DON'T that is often violated because we have always been told it is okay. Never eat an animal protein and a starchy vegetable or grain in the same meal. When you eat animal proteins, like eggs, meat, poultry, or fish, your stomach produces hydrochloric acid and an enzyme called pepsin to digest them in the ideal, highly acidic condition. When you eat a starchy vegetable, like sweet potato or grain-like seeds, an enzyme called ptyalin is secreted, which develops an alkaline condition, because that is what is ideal for these foods to digest properly. Based on what we have already said about chemistry, can you see the problem?

Eating animal proteins and starches or grains together means the acid and alkali neutralize each other, enzymes can't do their jobs, digestion stalls, and your food begins to ferment. This is feast time for pathogenic bacteria and yeast, like Candida, that are in your digestive tract.

Think of the typical North American diet—ham or turkey sandwiches, steak and baked potato, pizza, burgers and fries. These combinations all have protein and starch in the same meal, which is a big no-no in the food-combining world. You may be wondering, "What can I eat then, if I can't eat the typical North American diet?" You can eat lots of food, actually. You just have to make sure you follow the rules. At first, food-combining may seem complicated, but I promise you once you get a handle on it, it will be like second nature to you. Your digestive tract has taken assault after assault, and the Standard American Diet (S.A.D.) makes it obvious why food allergies, food sensitivity, food intolerance, obesity, and other illnesses are at epidemic levels. These diseases will continue to rise unless we start changing the way we think about the food on our plates. Sadly, the Western diet has already been proven to change gut bacteria and trigger the development of more serious gastric diseases, including colitis. Eating Western foods may even increase the risk of death.

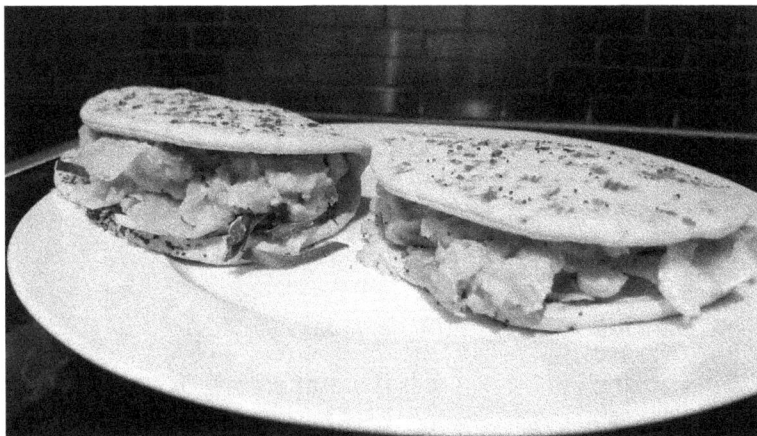

These avocado sandwiches demonstrate the food combining method by combining starch with vegetables, which is an excellent combination.

FOOD-COMBINING RULES EXPLAINED: DIGESTIVE PRINCIPLES CANNOT BE SEPARATED

All of your organs work together in harmony to create balance in your inner system, and takes you towards better health. You cannot practice one and ignore the others.

Principles of 80/20 for a Small Waist

- *Principle #1 – Eat Until 80% Full, Leaving 20% Room for Digestion*

  Overeating is always bad news for your stomach. When you overeat, you create high residue. Undigested food ferments and not only creates misery in the form of gas, bloating, and constipation, but also feeds opportunistic organisms. If you leave 20% room for digestive juices to work their magic, you will be more balanced.

- *Principle #2 – Eat 80% Vegetables and 20% Other*

  'Other' includes animal proteins OR grains, like millet, amaranth, quinoa, buckwheat, OR starches, like rice, potatoes, squash, beans.

- *Principle #3 – Eat 80% Alkaline and 20% Acidic*

  If you eat 80% vegetables with every meal, you will follow this principle. If you drink quality water or herbal teas all day long, and avoid acidic beverages, such as pop and juices, it will help. Drinking vegetable juices that you juice yourself is very alkalizing and beneficial.

- *Principle #4 – Eat 80% Raw and 20% Cooked*

  Cooking vegetables kills the nutrients, so it's best to eat vegetables raw. This will allow your body to receive lots of nutrients from the food that you eat.

I also use the following tricks in conjunction with food-combining and the 80/20 rule. These tips are also on my website (www.dinewithabby.ca).

First tip: Drink lemon water mixed with 2 tablespoons of apple cider vinegar in the morning before eating breakfast. I drink this mixture throughout the day, and I also try to drink as much water as I can in a day, sometimes 1L, sometimes 2L. Each person requires a different amount of water each day.

Second tip: Waist trainer. I wear my waist trainer from the moment I wake up and take it off right before bedtime. I know some people may say, "Oh, it messes up your organs," but that is a misguided judgement. If that really was the case, I wouldn't have been able to successfully give birth to my fourth beautiful child. I have been waist training since 2013, so this I can tell you from my four years of experience, wearing a waist trainer for that long will not mess up your organs.

Third tip: Chlorella tablets. This tablet cleans you inside out. It makes you glow, gives you a youthful look, detoxifies, and so much more.

Fourth tip: I eat a bunch of fruits on an empty stomach for breakfast. If I am having sweet fruits, I stick to the sweet fruit category. If am eating fruits from the acidic category, I stick to the acidic category, and the same for the sub-acidic fruits. I follow the food-combining rule, and I refer to the chart to see what food goes with what when I am not sure.

Fifth tip: When making smoothies, I don't use dairy. I use almond milk. In addition, I add chia seeds, hemp seeds, pumpkin seeds, and almonds, depending on the type of smoothie I am making.

Sixth tip: I hardly drink alcohol, and I don't smoke at all. If you do drink alcohol or smoke, I would just recommend minimizing however much of it you consume by half, and then slowly reducing that. This would be the best option to increase your health and minimize, or remove completely, addictive side effects. I only have one body, so my goal is to make it last for the rest of my life.

Seventh tip: Exercise. I train with my significant other, Wayne from BuffBoy Fitness, whenever the baby allows me to. Exercise doesn't have to be an extreme thing every morning and night. Even a walk every morning is the beginning to a healthier body.

Eighth tip: Get rid of whatever and whoever may be stressing you out. Life is short, so it is very important to live it to the fullest.

Things to remember:

- Always eat fruit alone on an empty stomach.

- Avoid combining proteins (beans, nuts, meat) with carbs (pasta, bread, starch, grains).

- Save protein, heavier foods, and cheat foods for the last meal of the day.

- Wait three hours after eating a grain-based meal before you have a protein meal.

- After a protein meal, give yourself four hours to fully digest.

- Stevia can be used as a calorie-free natural sugar substitute to satisfy sugar cravings.

- Try not to drink cold water during meals. Drink a big glass of water thirty minutes before each meal. This will super-hydrate your stomach, encouraging it to produce more hydrochloric acid, and increasing the flow of bile and pancreatic enzymes.

- A cup of warm tea, or room temperature water, will aid digestion, but drink it one hour after eating.

- Avoid ice when you drink water. Stick to room temperature water that doesn't shock your body, and do not drink for at least fifteen minutes before you eat, or one hour after a meal.

- Remember, it's never too late to change your life.

Follow these tips, and you can be sure your waist, body, and mental health will be transformed.

FOOD COMBINING CHART

Proper food combining not only helps with transforming your waist, it also gives you great skin and renewed energy.

Average Food Digestion Times

- Water: 15 minutes
- Melon: 1 hour
- Fruits: 1-2 hours
- Vegetables: 2.5 hours
- Fat: 3 hours
- Starch: 3 hours
- Protein: 4+ hours

- Melons are best eaten on their own because it digests pretty fast
- Eat fruits on an empty stomach or as a stand alone meal
- Eat only one type of concentrated starch or protein at a time because each protein has its own gastric juice, timing, and enzyme needed
- Wait 3 to 4 hours before switching between protein and starch
- Drink water 1 hour after eating. DO NOT DRINK COLD WATER WHILE YOU'RE EATING. It will slow down the digestion of the food
- Stay away from dairy
- Netrual foods can be combined with anything
- Avocado combines well with all foods except protein and melons
- Tomato is an acid fruit so it can be combined with non-starchy vegetables

Excellent Combos

- Non-Starchy Vegetables and Starchy
- Non-Starchy Vegetables and Protein
- Non-Starchy Vegetables and Mildly-Starchy Vegetables
- Non-Starchy Vegetables and Fats and Oils
- Sub-Acid Fruits and Acid Fruits

Bad Combos

- Protein and Starch together in a meal
- Protein and Fats and Oils
- Protein and Sugar
- Starch and Sugar
- Starch and Acid
- Acid Fruits and Sweet Fruits
- Acid Fruits and Fats and Oils
- Sweet Fruits and Starches

Neutral Foods
can be combined with any food

- Coconut Water
- Almond Milk
- Dark Chocolate
- Raw, Leafy Greens
- Herbs and Seasoning
- Seed oils

Protein

- Seafood
- Meat
- Nuts
- Seeds
- Eggs
- Cheese
- Yogurt
- Chicken

Melons

- Cantaloupe
- Casaba
- Honey Dew
- Watermelon

Fats and Oils

- Butter
- Creams
- Ghee
- Canola Oil
- Vegetable Oil

Starch

- Potatoes
- Breads
- Grains
- Beans
- Cereals
- Squash
- Pumpkin

Acid Fruits

- Sour Apples
- Grapes
- Lemons
- Cranberries
- Oranges
- Pineapples
- Strawberries
- Tomatoes
- Pomegranates

Sub-Acid Fruits

- Apples
- Apricots
- Blueberries
- Cherries
- Mangoes
- Peaches
- Pears
- Plums
- Guava

Sweet Fruits

- Bananas
- Dates
- Currants
- Figs
- Papayas
- Persimmons
- Prunes
- Raisins
- Dried Fruits

Starchy Vegetables

- Sweet Potatoes
- Yams
- Beans
- Jicamas
- Summer Squash

Mildly Starchy Vegetables

- Peas
- Carrots
- Cauliflowers
- Corn
- Beets
- Artichokes

Non-Starchy Vegetables

- Leafy Greens
- Onions
- Mushrooms
- Scallions
- Sweet Peppers
- Garlic
- Eggplant
- Brussel Sprouts
- Ginger
- Celery
- Zucchini
- Radishes
- Cucumber
- Sprouts
- Turnips
- Asparagus
- Beet Greens
- Broccoli
- Leeks
- Green Beans

The secret of getting ahead is getting started.

MARK TWAIN

CHAPTER 5
Recipes and Menu Samples

I don't know about you, but whenever I buy a book that has recipes in the back, 95% of the time, I don't follow the recipes, because they ask for lots of ingredients, or the ingredients are not available at my local grocery store, or they take too long to make. I am a mother of four, so time is something I have to spend wisely. I don't have all day to be making food with complicated recipes that take too long to prepare. The recipes that are included in this chapter take only thirty minutes or less to prepare.

The following are breakfast, lunch, dinner, and snack recipes using the food-combining method.

BREAKFAST

Pine-Straw Smoothie

- 2 cups of coconut water
- 1 cup of strawberries
- 1 cup of pineapple chunks
- 4–5 ice cubes (optional)

Directions
1. Combine all ingredients in a blender and blend.
2. Enjoy.

Avocado Smoothie

- 2 cups of almond or coconut milk
- 1 avocado
- 1 cup of grapes (seedless)

Directions
1. Combine ingredients in a blender and blend.
2. Enjoy.

Pineapple Smoothie

- 1 cup of coconut water
- 1 cup of pineapple chunks

Directions
1. Combine ingredients in a blender and blend.
2. Enjoy.

Spinach Muffin

- 2 cups of fresh or frozen spinach
- 5 eggs
- 1 garlic clove minced
- Pinch of nutmeg
- ½ tsp paprika
- Salt and pepper to taste

Directions
1. Preheat oven to 360°F
2. Lightly grease the muffin cups with coconut oil
3. In a large bowl, whip the eggs and spices until blended
4. Fold in spinach, then spoon mixture into muffin cups
5. Bake for 20 minutes or until the egg has formed

Spi-Ban Smoothie

- 1 cup of almond milk
- 1 banana
- 2 cups of spinach
- 3 ice cubes (optional)

Directions
1. Pour the almond milk into the blender first, and then add the rest of the ingredients.
2. Blend until smooth.
3. Enjoy!

Aloe Vera Smoothie

- ¼ cup of frozen mango chunks
- ¾ cup of fresh pineapple chunks
- ½ cup of aloe vera juice
- ¼ cup of cashew milk

Directions

1. Combine all ingredients in a blender and blend until smooth.
2. Add more milk or juice as needed to thin the smoothie to the desired consistency. Enjoy!

_____

In case you are thinking, "If I can't eat eggs and toast together, then what can I do?" this recipe is for you.

Bell Pepper Eggs

- 1 red bell pepper (yellow works just as well)
- 4–5 large eggs
- Salt
- Pepper
- Parsley flakes
- 1 tbsp of coconut oil

Directions

1. In a large pan, heat 1 tbsp of coconut oil over medium/high heat.
2. Cut peppers into ½ inch rings and remove the seeds and centres.
3. Place sliced peppers into the pan and let them sauté for a minute.
4. Crack each egg and slowly pour it into the centre of each bell pepper slice. Pouring the egg in slowly will prevent it from leaking.
5. Sprinkle salt, pepper, and parsley over each egg. Sauté for 3 minutes, then flip it over carefully.
6. Cook for another minute, then serve.

_____

Mango-Peach Smoothie

- 2 cups of coconut milk
- 1 cup of mango chunks
- 1 cup of peach chunks
- 1 cup of kale

Directions
1. Combine all ingredients in a blender and blend.
2. Enjoy.

Blueberry Smoothie

- ½ cup of coconut yogurt* (recipe located in the Snack section)
- ½ cup of frozen blueberries
- ½ cup of frozen pineapple
- 1 cup of kale
- ¾ cup of water

Directions
1. Combine all ingredients in a blender and blend.
2. Enjoy.

Papaya Smoothie

- 1 can of coconut water
- 2 cups of papaya
- ½ cup of spinach
- 2 dates
- Ice cubes (optional)

Directions
1. Combine all the ingredients in a blender and blend.
2. Enjoy.

LUNCH

Flax Egg

(substitute for egg in baking)
- 1 tbsp of ground flax or chia seeds
- 3 tbsp of water

Directions
1. Whisk together the ground seeds and water until well combined, then place in the fridge to set for 15 minutes.
2. Use as you would an egg in many of your favourite baking recipes.

Grilled Cheese Sandwich

(makes 2 sandwiches)

- 2 medium freshly shredded raw zucchini
- 2 tbsp of ground flax seed
- 6 tbsp of water
- ¾ cup of all-purpose flour
- ½ tsp of salt
- ¼ tsp of ground black pepper
- 2 thick slices of cheese of your choice

Directions
1. Preheat oven to 400°F.
2. Line a large baking sheet with parchment paper.
3. Add shredded zucchini to a large bowl and let sit 10-15 minutes, then drain excess water from zucchini bowl.
4. Add ½ cup of zucchini into a tea towel or paper towel and wring dry. Repeat with remaining zucchini.
5. Add in flax eggs, flour, salt, and pepper. Mix until all ingredients are thoroughly combined.
6. Divide zucchini batter evenly into four servings and place on baking sheet lined with parchment paper. Using a spatula, thin and spread out the divided batter to form four bread-square slices.
7. Bake in oven for about 15 minutes or until surface starts to turn a

light brown. Gently, using a spatula, flip breads over and cook for an additional 10 minutes or until the tops of the breads are a light brown.

8. Remove from oven and flip breads again. The side on top should now be crispy. The underside will be slightly softer, but this will be the inner bread sections where you will place the cheese.

9. Place one thick cheese slice in between two zucchini breads.

10. You can then cook these the traditional way, spreading some coconut oil on the outer bread surfaces and heating them on a skillet until cheese is melted, or you can microwave to melt the cheese.

Hash Brown

- 2 cups of cooked & shredded spaghetti squash (about ½ small cooked squash)
- 1 tbsp of coconut oil

Directions

1. Heat the oil in a large non-stick skillet over medium heat.
2. Press the water out of the squash with paper towels.
3. Form little patties by pressing the squash firmly between your palms.
4. Place the patties gently on the warmed skillet and let cook for 5-7 minutes per side. Only flip these once if possible to get the nice browned effect.
5. Transfer to paper towels to drain, then serve warm with any choice of sauce.

Quinoa Bowl

- 2 cups of cooked quinoa
- ½ cup of chopped yellow pepper
- 2 tbsp of parsley flakes
- 1 cup of chopped red pepper
- 1 Roma tomato

Dressing
- 2 tbsp of apple cider vinegar
- ¼ tbsp of olive oil
- Salt and pepper to taste

Directions
1. Add quinoa, bell peppers, tomato, and parsley flakes to a large bowl.
2. Whisk together the dressing ingredients in a separate small bowl.
3. Pour the dressing over the quinoa bowl and toss together.
4. Serve and enjoy.

Tomato-Avocado Salad
- 2 cups of diced Roma tomatoes (about 5)
- 1 zucchini
- ½ of medium red onion, sliced (optional)
- 2 avocados, diced
- 2 tbsp of extra virgin olive oil
- Juice of 1 medium lemon (about 2 tbsp)
- ¼ cup (½ bunch) parsley, chopped
- 1 tsp of sea salt

Directions
1. Place chopped tomatoes, sliced cucumber, sliced red onion, diced zucchini, and chopped parsley into a large salad bowl.
2. Drizzle with 2 tbsp olive oil, lemon juice, and salt.
3. Toss gently to combine.
4. Serve and enjoy.

Zucchini Fritters
- 2 cup shredded zucchini
- 2 scallions
- 2 large eggs
- ¼ cup of almond flour
- Salt and pepper to taste

Directions
1. Preheat oven 350°F
2. In a large bowl, combine zucchini, eggs, scallions, and almond flour
3. Season with salt and pepper
4. Form into fritter shapes and place in greased pan, or line the pan with parchment paper, and bake for 20 minutes.

Baked Cubes

- 2 cups of diced sweet potatoes
- 1 cup of diced carrots
- 2 tbsp of olive oil
- ½ tsp of salt
- 1 tsp of honey
- 2 tsp of Dijon mustard
- 2 tsp of chopped, curled parsley

Directions
1. Preheat oven 425°F.
2. Combine oil with salt in a large bowl.
3. Add sweet potato and carrot cubes, and stir until fully coated.
4. Put cubes on a pre-greased pan.
5. Roast in oven for 20 minutes, or until soft
6. In a small bowl, combine honey, Dijon mustard, and parsley.
7. Pour sauce over cooked cubes and serve.

Veggie Wrap

- 3 zucchinis, finely chopped
- ½ of a red onion, finely chopped
- 3 cloves of garlic, finely chopped
- ½ of a small jalapeno, seeded and finely chopped
- 2 tbsp of olive oil for sautéing
- ¼ tsp of sea salt
- ¼ tsp of chili powder
- ¼ tsp of cumin

- 2 cans of black beans, drained and well-rinsed

Toppings:
- 6 lettuce leaves for the wrap
- Guacamole or avocado
- Dulse flakes

Directions
1. Add the zucchini, garlic, onion, olive oil, and spices to a pan and cook for about 10-15 minutes over medium heat, stirring often.
2. Add the black beans to a separate frying pan and heat thoroughly over medium heat, stirring and mashing.
3. Place guacamole or avocado onto the lettuce, the heated beans, and cooked zucchini. Sprinkle the dulse and wrap everything with the lettuce leaf.

3-C Salad
- 2 cups of cauliflower florets
- 1 cucumber
- 1 can of drained corn
- ½ of a red pepper
- 3 green onions
- ½ cup of hummus
- Salt and pepper to taste

Directions
1. Cut the cauliflower into small florets.
2. Slice cucumber into thin slices.
3. Slice the red pepper and chop the green onions.
4. In a large bowl, combine the cauliflower, cucumber, red pepper, corn and green onions.
5. Add hummus, salt, and pepper, and mix well.
6. Serve and enjoy.

Coleslaw

- 1 cup of shredded cabbage
- 1 cup of shredded carrots
- ½ of a ripe avocado
- 1 tbsp of honey
- 1 lemon or lime, juiced
- Salt and pepper to taste

Directions

1. Whisk together all the ingredients, except the cabbage and carrots.
2. Toss in the cabbage and carrots, and mix together.
3. Serve and enjoy.

Beauty Salad

- 1 medium cucumber, diced
- 2 medium yellow peppers
- 2 cups of grape tomatoes, halved
- 1 cup of spinach

Dressing

- ¾ cup of coconut yogurt
- 1 tbsp of lemon juice
- 1 tbsp of olive oil

Directions

1. Whisk together yogurt, olive oil, and lemon juice in a small bowl.
2. Put remaining ingredients in a large bowl; spoon on dressing and toss to coat.
3. Serve and enjoy.

DINNER

Barbeque Meat and Rice

For Rice

- 3 cups of cauliflower
- 1 cup of broccoli, chopped
- 2-3 tbsp of water
- ¼ tsp of garlic salt
- 2 tbsp coconut oil
- 2 tsp lemon zest
- ½ of an onion
- 1 garlic clove, minced

Directions

1. Cut the hard core and stalks from the cauliflower.
2. Combine all the ingredients in a food processor or blender and pulse to make grains the size of rice.
3. Put into a heatproof bowl, and microwave for 7 minutes on High.

For Barbeque Meat

- 2 cans of young green jackfruit in water (Not in syrup or brine)
- ¼ cup of homemade barbeque sauce (2 tbsp cane sugar + 1 tsp onion powder + 1 tsp garlic powder + ½ tsp salt + ½ tsp pepper + ½ tsp chili powder)
- ¾ cup of barbeque sauce, any brand will do

Directions

1. Rinse, drain, and thoroughly dry jackfruit.
2. Chop off the centre 'core' portion of the fruit and discard. Place in a mixing bowl and set aside.
3. Mix together barbeque seasoning and add to jackfruit. Toss to coat.
4. Heat a large skillet over medium heat. Once hot, add 1-2 tbsp of coconut oil and seasoned jackfruit. Toss to coat, and cook for 2-3 minutes to achieve some colour.
5. Add barbeque sauce, then thin mixture with enough water to make it a sauce.
6. Reduce heat to low-medium, remove lid, stir occasionally, and cook for about 20 minutes.
7. Put the 'jack-meat' sauce on the bed of cauliflower rice. Enjoy.

Note: You can also use the jack-meat in a wrap or add it to a sandwich.

Baked Chicken

- 1 large chicken breast
- 1 bag of frozen Brussels sprouts
- 12 sticks of thin asparagus
- 2 tbsp of olive oil
- Garlic salt, salt, and pepper to taste

Directions

1. Place the chicken breast in the middle of a baking dish.
2. Cook sprouts as directed on the package.
3. Once they are cooked, lay them on one side of the chicken.
4. Place the raw asparagus on the other side of the chicken. Drizzle olive oil over both vegetables and sprinkle with garlic salt.
5. Sprinkle the chicken with salt, pepper, and garlic salt.
6. Bake at 400°F for 20 minutes.

Veggie Burger

- 1 cup of sliced mushrooms
- 1 medium shredded zucchini
- 1 cup of shredded carrots
- 2 tbsp of coconut oil
- 1 tbsp of grated ginger
- 3 tbsp of shredded scallion
- Salt, pepper, and cumin to taste

Directions

1. Combine all ingredients, except coconut oil, in a large bowl.
2. Shape into burger patties.
3. Add the coconut oil to skillet.
4. Cook the patties over medium heat until brown.

Note: You can serve this with sweet potato fries and use a lettuce leaf as the bun.

Zucchini-Quinoa

- 1 ¼ cup of coconut milk
- 2 cups of cooked quinoa
- 2 cups of chopped yellow peppers
- 2 cups of chopped Zucchini
- 2 tbsp of olive oil
- Salt and pepper to taste

Directions

1. Toss the cooked quinoa in 1 tbsp of olive oil.
2. In a large frying pan, sauté bell peppers for 1 minute in 1 tbsp of oil.
3. Add zucchini and sauté for 2 minutes.
4. Add coconut milk and simmer for 5 minutes.
5. Add salt and pepper to taste.
6. Add quinoa to the sauce and toss.
7. Serve and enjoy.

Spaghetti Squash

- 1 (2-3lb) spaghetti squash
- 2 tbsp of olive oil
- 1 tbsp of coconut oil
- 1 onion
- 2 cups of sliced mushrooms
- 2 cups of low fat table cream
- Sea salt and freshly ground black pepper to taste

Directions

1. Preheat oven to 375° F.
2. Lightly grease a baking sheet or coat with non-stick spray.
3. Put squash in microwave for 5 minutes. It makes it easier to cut.
4. Cut the squash in half, lengthwise from stem to tail, and scrape out the seeds.
5. Drizzle with olive oil and season with salt and pepper to taste.
6. Place squash cut-side down onto the prepared baking dish.
7. Put into oven and roast until tender, about 20-35 minutes.
8. While the squash is in the oven, add 1 tbsp of coconut oil to a

frying pan
9. Add onion, and cook for 1 minute
10. Add garlic and mushroom, and cook for 3 minutes
11. Add table cream
12. Remove squash from oven and let rest until cool enough to handle. Using a fork, scrape the flesh to create long strands.
13. Put the sauce on the spaghetti and serve.

Sweet Potatoes

- 6 small sweet potatoes, peeled, quartered, and sliced
- 1 tsp of paprika
- 2 tsp of salt
- 1 tsp of pepper
- 2 tsp of garlic powder
- 1 tsp of ground cinnamon
- 2 tbsp of extra virgin olive oil
- Non-stick cooking spray

Directions
1. Preheat your oven to 450°F.
2. Pour the oil into a small bowl, then stir all the seasonings into the oil.
3. Place the sliced sweet potatoes into a large bowl.
4. Pour the seasoning mixture over the potatoes and, using tongs or your hands, evenly coat the potatoes.
5. Spray a large baking sheet with cooking spray.
6. Lay the sweet potatoes on the baking sheet, do not overlap.
7. Use the cooking spray to lightly coat the sweet potatoes.
8. Bake for 10 minutes, turn them, spray with cooking spray again, and bake for 10 more minutes until tender.
9. Cool for 5 minutes before serving.

Quinoa and Cheese

(remix version of Mac and Cheese)

- 1 box of quinoa pasta
- 2 tbsp of parsley flakes
- 1½ cups of cauliflower, chopped
- 1½ cups of sweet potato, diced
- 1 cup of nutritional yeast
- 1 cup of steamed broccoli
- ¾ cup of almond milk
- ¼ cup of olive oil
- 2 cloves of garlic
- 1 tsp of salt
- 1 tsp of onion powder
- 1 tsp of cumin

Directions
1. Bring water to a boil in a medium pot or steamer
2. Steam sweet potato, broccoli, and cauliflower until soft, about 10-15 minutes.
3. Cook pasta according to packet directions and drain.
4. While pasta is cooking, add everything except the pasta, broccoli, and parsley to a blender and blend until smooth
5. Combine cooked pasta, cheese sauce from blender, broccoli and parsley in a large bowl.
6. Toss together and serve.

Pesto Pizza
- 3 cups of cooked mashed butternut squash (1 large squash)
- 1 cup of almond flour
- ¾ cup of chick pea flour
- ¼ tsp of sea salt
- 1/8 tsp of black pepper
- 3 tbsp of ground flax
- 1 tsp of parsley flakes

Toppings:
- Pesto sauce* and topping of choice

Directions
1. Begin by preparing the squash for roasting. Cut the squash in half lengthwise, and scoop out the seeds. 2. Lay cut-side down in a roasting pan, and fill pan halfway with water. Cook in oven at 200°F for 40 minutes, or until a fork can easily pierce the flesh of the squash. Let cool, then scoop out the flesh.
2. In a small bowl, combine the 2 tbsp of ground flax with 4 tbsp of water, and let sit for 5 minutes.
3. In a large bowl, combine 3 cups of squash with the soaked flax meal, almond flour, chickpea flour, salt, pepper, dried oregano, and extra ground flax.
4. Stir to combine.
5. Spread the mixture onto a parchment lined tray and create a circle, making sure that the edges are a little bit thicker than the centre.
6. Bake in the oven at 220°F for 30 minutes, or until the edges are crisp and golden.
7. Top with pizza sauce and choice of vegetable toppings, and bake for another 10 minutes.
8. Enjoy.

*Pesto Sauce Recipe:
- ½ cup of packed basil
- 1 cup of packed spinach
- ½ lemon, juiced
- Sea salt and pepper to taste
- 8 tbsp of olive oil

Directions
1. In a food processor, puree the basil and spinach until smooth.
2. Add the salt, pepper, lemon juice, and oil, and mix to combine.

Okra Salmon

- 2 skinless salmon filets
- 2 small zucchinis, sliced into half moons
- 8 okras, sliced in half
- 2 shallots, 1 thinly sliced and 1 chopped
- 2 cloves of garlic, minced
- 2 ½ tbsp of olive oil, divided
- Salt and ground black pepper
- 2 tbsp of fresh lemon juice
- 1 tbsp of thyme
- ¾ tsp of dried oregano

Directions

1. Preheat oven to 400°F.
2. Cut 2 sheets of aluminum foil big enough to hold the salmon and veggies.
3. Toss zucchini, okra, sliced shallot, and garlic together with 1 tbsp of olive oil. Season with salt and pepper to taste.
4. Divide on 2 sheets of foil, placing veggies in the centre of the foil.
5. Brush salmon filets with 1 tbsp of olive oil, season bottom side with salt and pepper, then place one filet on top of each layer of veggies on foil.
6. Drizzle lemon juice over salmon, and season top with salt and pepper.
7. Toss remaining diced shallot, thyme, oregano with remaining 1 ½ tsp of olive oil, season lightly with salt and pepper, and divide the remaining shallot mixture over salmon fillets.
8. Wrap sides of foil inward, then fold ends to seal. Place on a rimmed baking sheet and bake in preheated oven until salmon is cooked through, about 25-30 minutes.

Broccoli Potatoes

- 4 large purple-skin sweet potatoes
- 2 cups of broccoli florets
- 3 tbsp of olive oil
- 2 cloves of garlic, minced
- 1 tbsp of cumin
- ¼ tsp of onion powder
- Salt and freshly ground black pepper, to taste
- 2 tbsp of chopped fresh parsley leaves

Directions

1. Preheat oven to 400°F.
2. Add the potatoes, broccoli florets, olive oil, garlic, cumin, and onion powder to a small bowl; whisk together and season with salt and pepper to taste.
3. Place into oven and bake until tender, about 12-14 minutes.
4. Sprinkle with parsley.
5. Serve and enjoy.

Homemade Tortillas

- 2 cups of all-purpose flour, or any other type of flour, except coconut flour (plus extra for kneading and dusting)
- ½ tsp of salt
- ¾ cup of water, room temperature
- 3 tbsp of olive oil or coconut oil

Directions

1. Combine 2 cups of flour and the salt in a food processor.
2. Combine the oil and water and drizzle it in.
3. Process until the dough comes together and forms a ball. (If you are using your hand, knead for at least 5 minutes, or until the dough is smooth.)
4. Turn the dough onto a floured surface and knead several times until the dough is smooth.
5. Form into a ball, cover with a towel, and let the dough rest for 15 minutes.

6. Preheat a cast-iron skillet, griddle, or frying pan over medium heat.
7. Divide the dough into eight portions and roll into balls.
8. On a lightly floured surface, flatten the balls and use a rolling pin to roll each ball into an 8-inch or 9-inch circle. Sprinkle with flour as needed to prevent sticking.
9. In the preheated skillet, cook tortillas over medium heat for about 30 to 45 seconds on each side or until light brown spots appear and the tortilla is puffy.
10. Transfer the tortillas to a plate and cover with a clean towel to keep warm.

Note: The tortillas can be packed with your favourite vegetables to make a wrap.

DETOXIFYING WATER

Detoxifying is a very important part of maintaining optimal health. We eat, breathe, and sleep chemicals in the modern world that we live in. These chemicals can wreak havoc on our health, so it is very important to get rid of the toxins from our bodies by detoxifying so we can be healthy and live a vibrant life.

Water is the best beverage that you can drink for your body. It hydrates you, detoxifies your body, and does many more amazing things. I don't know about you, but I get bored with drinking plain water, so I add different fruits and herbs to spruce up the taste. Below are different versions of water that I drink.

Drinking water throughout the day will improve digestion, and prevent cravings, constipation, and bloating.

Lemon Cucumber Water

- 2L of water
- 1 lemon, juiced
- ½ of a cucumber
- 12 mint leaves

Directions
1. Combine and sip throughout the day.

———————————————

Anti-Bloat Water

- 3L of water
- 2 tbsp of apple cider vinegar
- 12 parsley leaves
- 12 small mint leaves
- 1 tsp of freshly grated ginger
- 1 medium lemon, thinly sliced
- 1 medium cucumber, peeled and thinly sliced

Directions
1. Combine all the ingredients and let it sit overnight in the fridge.
2. Drink 8-10 glasses daily at room temperature.

———————————————

Berry and Parsley Water

- 2L of water
- 1 cup of your favourite berries
- 1 cup of parsley leaves

Directions
1. Combine ingredients and sip throughout the day.

———————————————

Strawberry-Lemon Water

- 2L of water
- 1 cup of sliced strawberries
- 1 lemon
- 12 mint leaves

Directions
1. Combine ingredients and sip throughout the day.

Orange Blueberry Water

- 2L of water
- 1 orange
- 1 cup of blueberries

Directions
1. Combine ingredients and sip throughout the day.

Pineapple-Mint Water

- 2L of water
- 1 cup of pineapples
- 12 mint leaves

Directions
1. Combine ingredients and sip throughout the day.

Cucumber-Mint Water

- 2L of water
- 1 cucumber, sliced in circles
- 13 mint leaves

Directions
1. Combine ingredients and sip throughout the day.

Citrus Water

- 2L of water
- 1 lime, cut in circles
- 1 orange, cut in circles
- 1 grapefruit, cut in circles
- 1 lemon, cut in circles

Directions
1. Combine ingredients and sip throughout the day.

Orange Kiwi Water

- 2L of water
- 1 orange, cut in circles
- 2 kiwis, peeled and cut in circles

Directions
1. Combine ingredients and sip throughout the day.

Lemon Ginger Water

- 2L of water
- Juice from 1 lemon
- 3 tbsp unfiltered apple cider vinegar
- 2-inch knob of ginger, sliced

Directions
1. Combine ingredients and sip throughout the day.

Raspberry Lemon Water

- 2L of water
- 1 cup of raspberries
- 1 lemon

Directions

1. Combine ingredients and sip throughout the day.

SNACKS

Vegan Caramel

(can be used as a fruit dip or caramel apple)

- 2 cups of pitted pre-soaked dates
- 8 tbsp of almond milk
- ½ tsp of sea salt
- 1/3 cup of coconut oil

Directions

1. Combine all ingredients in a food processor.
2. Blend and enjoy.

Flax Egg

(substitute for egg in baking)
- 1 tbsp of ground flax or chia seeds
- 3 tbsp of water

Directions

1. Whisk together the ground seeds and water until well combined, then place in the fridge to set for 15 minutes.
2. Use as you would an egg in many of your favourite baking recipes.

Squash Cake

(delicious)

- 2 cups of cooked spaghetti squash
- 1 cup of all-purpose flour
- 2 tsp of baking powder
- ¼ tsp of baking soda
- 1 tsp of cinnamon
- 1 tsp of ginger
- ½ tsp of cardamom
- ½ cup of honey
- ¼ cup of coconut oil
- 2 tbsp of grounded flax seed
- 6 tbsp of water

Directions

1. Preheat oven to 375°F.
2. Lightly grease a baking sheet, or coat with non-stick spray.
3. Put squash in microwave for 5 minutes, which makes it easier to cut.
4. Cut the squash in half lengthwise, from stem to tail, and scrape out the seeds.
5. Drizzle with olive oil.
6. Place squash, cut-side down, onto the prepared baking dish, then put into the oven and roast until tender, about 20-35 minutes.
7. Spray an 8x8inch baking pan with cooking spray and set aside.
8. In a small bowl, combine the flax seed and water to make the flax egg. Put into fridge for 15 minutes.
9. In a medium bowl, stir the flour, baking powder, baking soda, cinnamon, ginger, and cardamom together.
10. In another small bowl, whisk the maple syrup and coconut oil together.
11. Add in the flax egg and stir.
12. Mix the wet ingredients with the dry.
13. Fold in the squash.
14. Bake for 25-28 minutes, or until toothpick comes out clean.
15. Cool, serve and enjoy.

Mango Ice Cream

- 2 frozen bananas, cut in pieces
- ½ cup of frozen mango chunks

Directions

1. Combine in a blender and blend.
2. Serve and enjoy.

Blueberry Ice Cream

- 2 frozen bananas, cut in pieces
- ½ cup of frozen blueberries

Directions

1. Combine in a blender and blend.
2. Serve and enjoy.

Coconut Yogurt

- 2 (14 oz.) cans of additive-free coconut milk
- 2 probiotic capsules
- 2 tsp of agar or tapioca starch
- 2 tbsp of coconut sugar, organic sugar, or maple syrup

Directions

1. Dissolve agar or tapioca starch with coconut milk, and set aside in a 2 quart size mason jar.
2. Open the probiotic capsules and pour the probiotic culture into the coconut milk, and mix well.
3. Add the sugar, and mix well.
4. Put the sealed jar of yogurt in the oven with the light on. Do not turn the oven on. Just close the oven door and turn on the oven light. The closed oven and the light generate a stable temperature of about 105-110°F, which is perfect for incubating the coconut milk for 18-24 hours.

If you do not want to wait 18-24 hours, here is a quicker recipe:

- 1 young coconut or (frozen coconut meat) and can of coconut water
- 2 probiotic pills
- 2 tbsp of cane sugar

Directions
1. Cut open the young coconut and separate the meat. Blend the meat and water together in a blender. If using frozen meat and coconut water, just add both to the blender.
2. Pour the mixture into a bowl.
3. Open up the probiotic capsules and pour into the mixture.
4. Add 2 tbsp of sugar.
5. Serve and enjoy.

Note: Can be used as a snack or part of a salad dressing.

Chia Pudding
- 2 ½ cups of almond milk
- 3 tbsp of pure maple syrup
- ½ cup of chia seeds
- ¼ cup of walnuts, roasted

Directions
1. Add almond milk, maple syrup, and chia seeds to a jar and stir well.
2. Seal the jar, and refrigerate overnight.
3. Sprinkle walnuts on top in the morning and enjoy.

Plaintain Chips

- 1 medium ripe plantain
- 2 tbsp of coconut oil
- 2 tbsp of parsley flakes

Directions

1. Preheat the oven to 350°F.
2. Peel and slice the plantain in thin circles.
3. Place slices on a baking sheet lined with parchment paper.
4. Add the coconut oil and toss to coat plantain slices.
5. Place in oven and bake for 20 minutes.
6. Garnish with parsley flakes.

Broccoli Bites

- 2 cups of broccoli, cooked and chopped
- 1 egg

Directions

1. Preheat oven to 350°F.
2. Spray mini muffin tin with non-stick baking spray.
3. Combine broccoli and egg in a food processor or blender, and blend well.
4. Spoon mixture into a mini muffin tin until about ¾ full.
5. Bake at 350°F for 12-15 minutes.

No-Bake Brownies

- 2 cups of pre-soaked, pitted dates
- 1 cup of almond flour
- ½ cup of cocoa/cacao powder

Directions

1. Blend all the ingredients together in a food processor or blender until you get a doughy consistency.
2. Line a small baking sheet with parchment paper.
3. Pour the mixture onto the baking sheet.
4. Spread evenly with a spatula.
5. Freeze for 1 hour or put in the fridge for 2 hours.

———————————————

Date Bites

- 1 cup of presoaked, pitted dates
- ½ cup of almonds
- 2 tbsp of almond butter

Directions

1. Blend all ingredients together until you get a granola type texture.
2. Use your hand to form small balls.
3. Eat right away or save it for later.

———————————————

MEAL PLAN GROCERY LIST

The foods you will need for the next 30 days.

Fruits and Vegetables

Zucchini
Spaghetti Squash
Cucumber
Spinach
Parsley
Lemon
Mint
Berries (different types)
Banana
Granny Smith Apples
Papaya
Mangoes
Kiwi
Bell peppers
Oranges
Sweet Potatoes
Cauliflower
Broccoli
Plaintain
Okro
Jack fruit
Avocado
Onion
Celery
Dates
Grapefruit
Mushrooms
Corn
Tomatoes
Pineapples
Grapes
Cabbage
Carrots

Spices and Oils

Turmeric
Sea salt
Coconut oil
Olive oil
Black pepper
Ginger
Garlic
Cinnamon
Dried parsley

Nuts and seeds

Flax seed
Chia seed
Almond

Grains

Quinoa
Quinoa Spaghetti

Milk

Almond Milk
Coconut Milk
Cashew Milk

Condiments

Hummus
Honey
Vanilla extract
Apple cider Vinegar

Flour

All purpose flour
Coconut flour
Almond flour

Produce

Chicken
Fish
Eggs

MEAL PLAN: WEEK 1

Monday

Pre-Breakfast	30 minutes before breakfast, drink 1 glass of water with juice from ½ of a lemon and 2 tbsp of apple cider vinegar
Breakfast	Spi-Ban Smoothie
Snack	1 Granny Smith Apple with Vegan Caramel
Lunch	2 cups of Zucchini-Avocado Salad
Snack	2 cups of baby carrots with 2 tbsp of hummus
Dinner	Quinoa and Cheese
All Day	Sip 2L of your choice of detox water throughout the day.

Tuesday

Pre-Breakfast	30 minutes before breakfast, drink 1 glass of water with juice from ½ of a lemon and 2 tbsp of apple cider vinegar
Breakfast	Pine-Straw Smoothie
Snack	1 cup of Coconut Yogurt
Lunch	2 cups of Coleslaw
Snack	2 sliced red peppers and 2 tbsp of hummus
Dinner	Veggie Burger with lettuce bun
All Day	Sip 2L of your choice of detox water throughout the day.

MEAL PLAN: WEEK 1

Wednesday

Pre-Breakfast	30 minutes before breakfast, drink 1 glass of water with juice from ½ of a lemon and 2 tbsp of apple cider vinegar
Breakfast	Avocado Smoothie
Snack	1 cup of Chia Pudding with walnuts
Lunch	Zucchini Fritters
Snack	3 stalks of celery with 2 tbsp of hummus
Dinner	Sweet Potatoes
All Day	Sip 2L of your choice of detox water throughout the day.

Thursday

Pre-Breakfast	30 minutes before breakfast, drink 1 glass of water with juice from ½ of a lemon and 2 tbsp of apple cider vinegar
Breakfast	3 Spinach Muffins with 3 lettuce leaves
Snack	1 cup of Coconut Yogurt
Lunch	3-C Salad
Snack	2 cups of cauliflower florets with 2 tbsp of hummus
Dinner	Tortilla Wrap with veggie toppings of choice
All Day	Sip 2L of your choice of detox water throughout the day.

MEAL PLAN: WEEK 1

Friday

Pre-Breakfast	30 minutes before breakfast, drink 1 glass of water with juice from ½ of a lemon and 2 tbsp of apple cider vinegar
Breakfast	Mango-Peach Smoothie
Snack	1 cup of Blueberry Ice Cream
Lunch	Quinoa Bowl
Snack	1 cup of Chia Pudding with strawberry on top
Dinner	Spaghetti Squash
All Day	Sip 2L of your choice of detox water throughout the day.

Saturday

Pre-Breakfast	30 minutes before breakfast, drink 1 glass of water with juice from ½ of a lemon and 2 tbsp of apple cider vinegar
Breakfast	3 Bell Pepper Eggs
Snack	1 cup of Chia Pudding with crushed almonds
Lunch	Baked Cubes
Snack	2 cups of baby carrots with 2 tbsp hummus
Dinner	Zucchini Quinoa
All Day	Sip 2L of your choice of detox water throughout the day.

MEAL PLAN: WEEK 1

Sunday

Pre-Breakfast   30 minutes before breakfast, drink 1 glass of water
with juice from ½ of a lemon and 2 tbsp of apple
cider vinegar

Cheat Day

All Day   Sip 2L of your choice of detox water throughout
the day.

MEAL PLAN: WEEK 2

Monday

Pre-Breakfast	30 minutes before breakfast, drink 1 glass of water with juice from ½ of a lemon and 2 tbsp of apple cider vinegar
Breakfast	Aloe Vera Smoothie
Snack	1 cup of Coconut Yogurt
Lunch	Veggie Wrap
Snack	1 cup of broccoli florets with 2 tbsp hummus
Dinner	Barbecue Meat and Rice
All Day	Sip 2L of your choice of detox water throughout the day.

Tuesday

Pre-Breakfast	30 minutes before breakfast, drink 1 glass of water with juice from ½ of a lemon and 2 tbsp of apple cider vinegar
Breakfast	Papaya Smoothie
Snack	1 Granny Smith apple with 2 tbsp of Vegan Caramel
Lunch	Beauty Salad with Dressing
Snack	Plantain Chips
Dinner	Pesto Pizza
All Day	Sip 2L of your choice of detox water throughout the day.

MEAL PLAN: WEEK 2

Wednesday

Pre-Breakfast	30 minutes before breakfast, drink 1 glass of water with juice from ½ of a lemon and 2 tbsp of apple cider vinegar
Breakfast	Pineapple Smoothie
Snack	Mango Ice Cream
Lunch	Hash Brown with any choice of sauce
Snack	Broccoli Bites
Dinner	Baked Chicken
All Day	Sip 2L of your choice of detox water throughout the day.

Thursday

Pre-Breakfast	30 minutes before breakfast, drink 1 glass of water with juice from ½ of a lemon and 2 tbsp of apple cider vinegar
Breakfast	Blueberry Smoothie
Snack	2 slices of Squash Cake
Lunch	Grilled Cheese Sandwich
Snack	Plantain Chips
Dinner	Barbecue Meat and Rice
All Day	Sip 2L of your choice of detox water throughout the day.

MEAL PLAN: WEEK 2

Friday

Pre-Breakfast	30 minutes before breakfast, drink 1 glass of water with juice from ½ of a lemon and 2 tbsp of apple cider vinegar
Breakfast	1 grapefruit and 1 orange
Snack	No-Bake Brownie
Lunch	Veggie Wrap
Snack	2 slices of Squash Cake
Dinner	Okra Salmon
All Day	Sip 2L of your choice of detox water throughout the day.

Saturday

Pre-Breakfast	30 minutes before breakfast, drink 1 glass of water with juice from ½ of a lemon and 2 tbsp of apple cider vinegar
Breakfast	3 cups of mixed blueberry, strawberry, and black-berries
Snack	Date Bites
Lunch	3-C Salad
Snack	Plantain Chips
Dinner	Broccoli Potatoes
All Day	Sip 2L of your choice of detox water throughout the day.

MEAL PLAN: WEEK 2

Sunday

Pre-Breakfast   30 minutes before breakfast, drink 1 glass of water with juice from ½ of a lemon and 2 tbsp of apple cider vinegar

Cheat Day

All Day   Sip 2L of your choice of detox water throughout the day.

———————————————

MEAL PLAN: WEEK 3

Follow plan for Week 1.

———————————————

MEAL PLAN: WEEK 4

Follow plan for Week 2.

30 DAY SMALL WAIST EXERCISE PLAN

Day 1

45 sit ups

Day 2

30 sec side plank (both sides)
50 sit ups
50 leg raises

Day 3

35 side plank (both sides)
55 sit ups
55 leg raises

Day 4

40 sec plank
60 sit ups
60 leg raises

Day 5

Rest

Day 6

65 Crunches
65 leg raises

Day 7

Rest

Day 8

45 sec plank
70 leg raises
70 sit ups

Day 9

Rest

Day 10

30 squats
75 sit ups
30 sec plank

Day 11

40 sec side plank (both sides)
80 sit ups
40 squats

Day 12

30 Lunges
85 sit up
30 sec plank

Day 13

35 Lunges
45 squats
45 sec plank

Day 14

Rest

Day 15

90 sit ups
75 leg raises
1 min plank

Day 16

80 leg raises
40 squats
1 min side plank (both sides)

Day 17

95 sit ups
45 squats
40 Russian twist

Day 18

45 Russian twist
85 leg raises
50 squats

Day 19

Rest

Day 20

50 Russian twist
100 sit ups
90 leg raises

Day 21

55 Squats
1 min side plank (both sides)
40 Lunges

Day 22

105 sit ups
55 Russian twist
50 Lunges

Day 23

95 leg raises
1 min plank
60 squats

Day 24

100 leg raises
65 squats
60 Russian twists

Day 25

Rest

Day 26

70 Squats
1 minute plank
65 Russian twist

Day 27

55 Lunges
75 squats
1 min plank

Day 28

80 Squats
100 sit ups
100 leg raises

Day 29

85 Squats
50 Lunges
2 sets of 35 Russian twist

Day 30

100 sit ups
2 sets of 40 Russian twist
2 sets of 50 leg raises